The Inspired Diabetic Pressure Pot Cookbook

A Collection of Delicious Diabetic Pressure Pot Recipes for Your Healthy Meals

Cassandra Lane

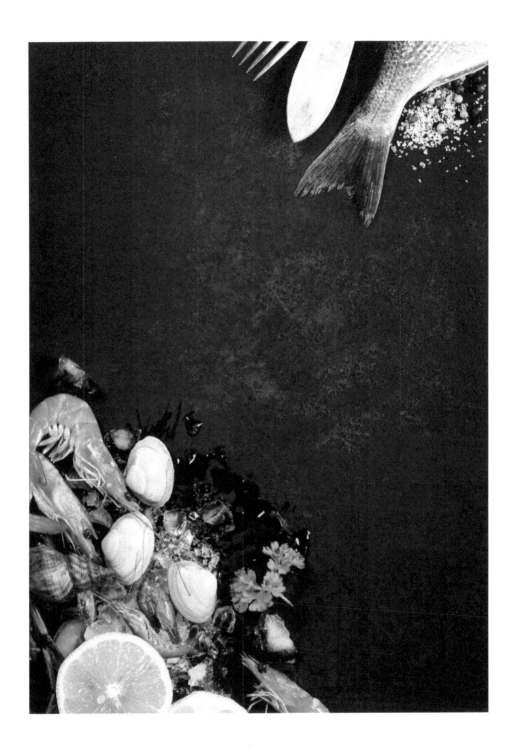

direct or indirect, which are incurred as a result of the use of information contained within this document, including, but not limited to, — errors, omissions, or inaccuracies.

Table of Contents

Salmon in Green Sauce

Servings: 4

Cooking Time: 12 Minutes

Ingredients:

• 4 (6-ounce) salmon fillets

• 1 avocado, peeled, pitted and chopped

• ½ cup fresh basil, chopped

• 3 garlic cloves, chopped

• 1 tablespoon fresh lemon zest, grated finely

Directions:

1. Grease a large piece of foil.

2. In a large bowl, add all ingredients except salmon and water and with a fork, mash completely.

3. Place fillets in the center of foil and top with avocado mixture evenly.

4. Fold the foil around fillets to seal them.

5. Arrange a steamer trivet in the Pressure Pot and pour ½ cup of water.

6. Place the foil packet on top of trivet.

7. Close the lid and place the pressure valve to "Seal" position.

8. Press "Manual" and cook under "High Pressure" for about minutes.

9. Meanwhile, preheat the oven to broiler.

10.Press "Cancel" and allow a "Natural" release.

11. Open the lid and transfer the salmon fillets onto a broiler pan.

12. Broil for about 3-4 minutes.

13. Serve warm.

14. Nutrition Info: Per serving: Calories: 333, Fats: 20.3g, Carbs: 5.5g, Sugar: 0.4g, Proteins: 34.2g, Sodium: 79mg

Braised Shrimp

Servings: 4

Cooking Time: 4 Minutes

Ingredients:

• 1 pound frozen large shrimp, peeled and deveined

• 2 shallots, chopped

• ¾ cup low-sodium chicken broth

• 2 tablespoons fresh lemon juice

• 2 tablespoons olive oil

• 1 tablespoon garlic, crushed

• Ground black pepper, as required

Directions:

1. In the Pressure Pot, place oil and press "Sauté". Now add the shallots and cook for about 2 minutes.

2. Add the garlic and cook for about 1 minute.

3. Press "Cancel" and stir in the shrimp, broth, lemon juice and black pepper.

4. Close the lid and place the pressure valve to "Seal" position.

5. Press "Manual" and cook under "High Pressure" for about 1 minute.

6. Press "Cancel" and carefully allow a "Quick" release.

7. Open the lid and serve hot.

8. Nutrition Info: Per serving: Calories: 209, Fats: 9g, Carbs: 4.3g, Sugar: 0.2g, Proteins: 26.6g, Sodium: 293mg

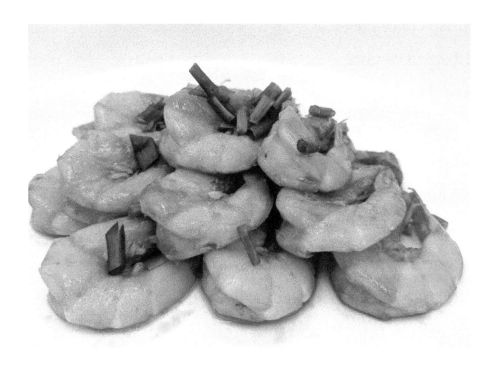

Shrimp Coconut Curry

Servings: 2

Cooking Time: 20 Minutes

Ingredients:

• 0.5lb cooked shrimp

• 1 thinly sliced onion

• 1 cup coconut yogurt

• 3tbsp curry paste

• 1tbsp oil or ghee

Directions:

1. Set the Pressure Pot to sauté and add the onion, oil, and curry paste.

2. When the onion is soft, add the remaining ingredients and seal.

3. Cook on Stew for 20 minutes.

4. Release the pressure naturally.

5. Nutrition Info: Per serving: Calories: 380; Carbs: 13; Sugar: 4 ; Fat: 22 ;Protein: 40 ; GL: 14

Trout Bake

Servings: 2

Cooking Time: 35 Minutes

Ingredients:

• 1lb trout fillets, boneless

• 1lb chopped winter vegetables

• 1 cup low sodium fish broth

• 1tbsp mixed herbs

• sea salt as desired

Directions:

1. Mix all the ingredients except the broth in a foil pouch.

2. Place the pouch in the steamer basket your Pressure Pot.

3. Pour the broth into the Pressure Pot.

4. Cook on Steam for 35 minutes.

5. Release the pressure naturally.

6. Nutrition Info: Per serving: Calories: 310; Carbs: 14; Sugar: 2 ; Fat: 12 ; Protein: 40 ; GL: 5

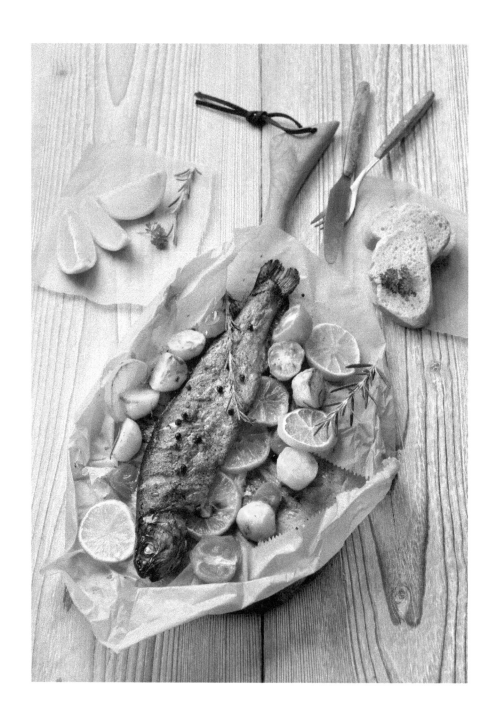

Sardine Curry

Servings: 2

Cooking Time: 35 Minutes

Ingredients:

• 5 tins of sardines in tomato

• 1lb chopped vegetables

• 1 cup low sodium fish broth

• 3tbsp curry paste

Directions:

1. Mix all the ingredients in your Pressure Pot.

2. Cook on Stew for 35 minutes.

3. Release the pressure naturally.

4. Nutrition Info: Per serving: Calories: 320; Carbs: 8; Sugar: 2 ; Fat: 16 ; Protein: ; GL: 3

Swordfish Steak

Servings: 2

Cooking Time: 35 Minutes

Ingredients:

• 1lb swordfish steak, whole

• 1lb chopped Mediterranean vegetables

• 1 cup low sodium fish broth• 2tbsp soy sauce

Directions:

1. Mix all the ingredients except the broth in a foil pouch.

2. Place the pouch in the steamer basket for your Pressure Pot.

3. Pour the broth into the Pressure Pot. Lower the steamer basket into the Pressure Pot.

4. Cook on Steam for 35 minutes.

5. Release the pressure naturally.

6. Nutrition Info: Per serving: Calories: 270; Carbs: 5; Sugar: 1 ; Fat: 10 ; Protein: 48 ; GL: 1

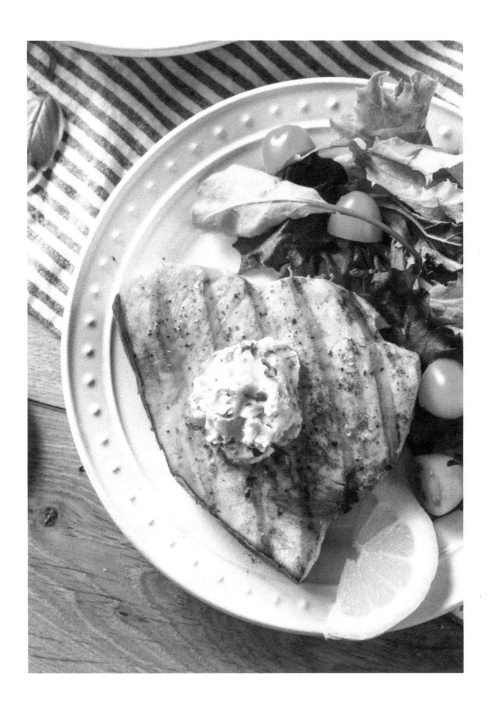

Lemon Sole

Servings: 2

Cooking Time: 5 Minutes

Ingredients:

• 1lb sole fillets, boned and skinned

• 1 cup low sodium fish broth

• 2 shredded sweet onions

• juice of half a lemon

• 2tbsp dried cilantro

Directions:

1. Mix all the ingredients in your Pressure Pot.

2. Cook on Stew for 5 minutes.

3. Release the pressure naturally.

4. Nutrition Info: Per serving: Calories: 230; Sugar: 1 ;

Fat: 6; Protein: 46 ; GL: 1

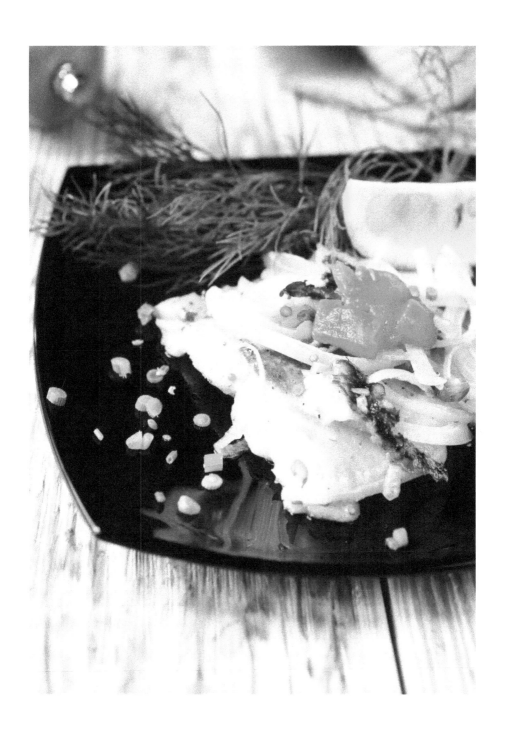

Trout Fillets Bake

Servings: 2

Cooking Time: 35 Minutes

Ingredients:

- 1 lb. trout fillets
- 1 lb. chopped winter vegetables
- 1 cup low sodium fish broth
- 1 tbsp. mixed herbs
- 1 tsp. Salt

Directions:

1. Mix all the ingredients except the broth in a foil pouch.
2. Place the pouch in the steamer basket your Pressure Pot.
3. Pour the broth into the Pressure Pot.
4. Cook on Steam for 35 minutes.
5. Release the pressure naturally.
6. Nutrition Info: Calories 310, Carbs 14g, Fat 12 g, Protein 40 g, Potassium (K) 335 mg, Sodium (Na) 229 mg

Tuna Sweetcorn Casserole

Servings: 2

Cooking Time: 35 Minutes

Ingredients:

• 3 small tins of tuna

• 0.5lb sweetcorn kernels

• 1lb chopped vegetables

• 1 cup low sodium vegetable broth

• 2tbsp spicy seasoning

Directions:

1. Mix all the ingredients in your Pressure Pot.

2. Cook on Stew for 35 minutes.

3. Release the pressure naturally.

4. Nutrition Info: Per serving: Calories: 300; Carbs: 6; Sugar: 1 ; Fat: 9 ; Protein: ; GL: 2

Chili Shrimp

Servings: 2

Cooking Time: 35 Minutes

Ingredients:

• 1.5lb cooked shrimp

• 1lb stir fry vegetables

• 1 cup ready-mixed fish sauce

• 2tbsp chili flakes

Directions:

1. Mix all the ingredients in your Pressure Pot.

2. Cook on Stew for 35 minutes.

3. Release the pressure naturally.

4. Nutrition Info: Per serving: Calories: 270; Carbs: 6; Sugar: ; Fat: 8 ;Protein: 51 ; GL: 2

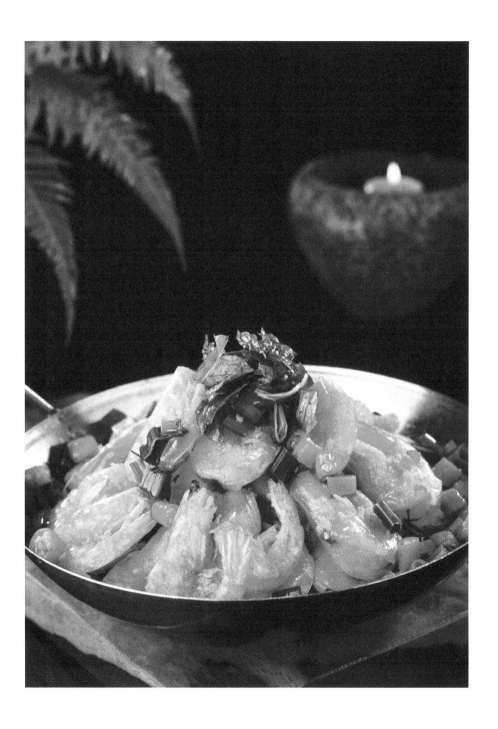

Lemon Pepper Salmon

Servings: 4

Cooking Time: 10 Minutes

Ingredients:

• 3 tbsps. ghee or avocado oil

• 1 lb. skin-on salmon filet

• 1 julienned red bell pepper

• 1 julienned green zucchini

• 1 julienned carrot

• ¾ cup water

• A few sprigs of parsley, tarragon, dill, basil or a combination

• ½ sliced lemon

• ½ tsp. black pepper

• ¼ tsp. sea salt

Directions:

1. Add the water and the herbs into the bottom of the Pressure Pot and put in a wire steamer rack making sure the handles extend upwards.

2. Place the salmon filet onto the wire rack, with the skin side facing down.

3. Drizzle the salmon with ghee, season with black pepper and salt, and top with the lemon slices.

4. Close and sealthe Pressure Pot, making sure the vent is turned to "Sealing".

5. Select the "Steam" setting and cook for 3 minutes.

6. While the salmon cooks, julienne the vegetables, and set aside.

7. Once done, quick release the pressure, and then press the "Keep Warm/Cancel" button.

8. Uncover and wearing oven mitts, carefully remove the steamer rack with the salmon.

9. Remove the herbs and discard them.

10. Add the vegetables to the pot and put the lid back on.

11.Select the "Sauté" function and cook for 1-2 minutes.

12. Serve the vegetables with salmon and add the remaining fat to the pot.

13. Pour a little of the sauce over the fish and vegetables if desired.

14. Nutrition Info: Calories 296, Carbs 8g, Fat 15 g,

Protein 31 g, Potassium (K) 1084 mg, Sodium (Na) 284 mg

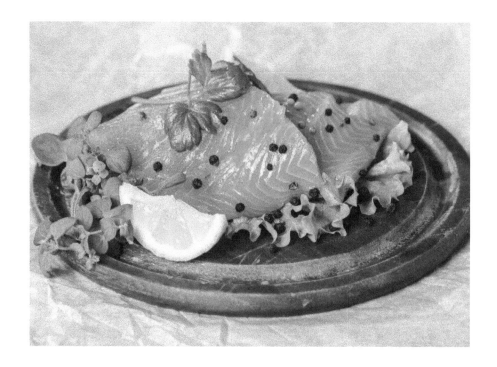

Mussels And Spaghetti Squash

Servings: 2

Cooking Time: 35 Minutes

Ingredients:

• 1lb cooked, shelled mussels

• 1/2 a spaghetti squash, to fit the Pressure Pot

• 1 cup low sodium fish broth

• 3tbsp crushed garlic

• sea salt to taste

Directions:

1. Mix the mussels with the garlic and salt. Place the mussels inside the squash.

2. Lower the squash into your Pressure Pot.

3. Pour the broth around it, cook on Stew for minutes.

4. Release the pressure naturally.

5. Shred the squash, mixing the "spaghetti" with the mussels.

6. Nutrition Info: Calories 2, Carbs 7g, Fat 9 g, Protein 24 g, Potassium (K) 124.8 mg, Sodium (Na) 462.6 mg

Cod in White Sauce

Servings: 2

Cooking Time: 5 Minutes

Ingredients:

• 1lb cod fillets

• 1lb chopped swede and carrots

• 2 cups white sauce

• 1 cup peas

• 3tbsp black pepper

Directions:

1. Mix all the ingredients in your Pressure Pot.

2. Cook on Stew for 5 minutes.

3. Release the pressure naturally.

4. Nutrition Info: Per serving: Calories: 390; Carbs: 10; Sugar: 2 ; Fat: 26 ; Protein: ; GL: 5

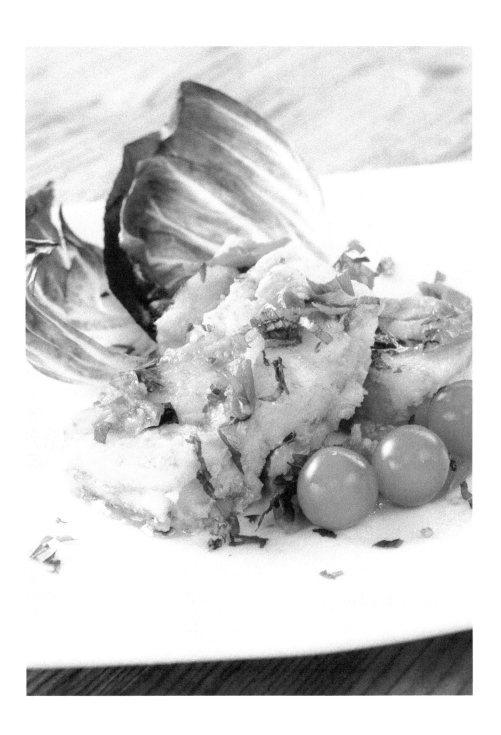

Lemon Pepper and Dill Salmon

Servings: 4

Cooking Time: 5 Minutes

Ingredients:

• 2 tbsp. Butter

• 1 lb. salmon filet

• 1 sliced lemon

• 3 thyme sprigs

• 1 fresh dill sprig

• 1 tsp. chopped dill

• Juice of 1 lemon

• Zest of 1 lemon

• 1 tsp. sea salt

• ¼ tsp. black pepper

Directions:

1. Add the butter, lemon zest, lemon juice, dill, salt, and pepper to a small mixing bowl. Mix well to form a compound butter.

2. Cut salmon into portion sizes, and place dollops of the compound butter all around the salmon portions.

3. Pour a cup of water into the Pressure Pot, along with

some thyme and/or dill.

4. Place half of the salmon onto a standard trivet and insert this into the pot.

5. Season with more pepper, and then top the fish with 2 thin slices of lemon.

6. Place the second half of the fish onto a 3-inch trivet and insert into the pot. Season with more black pepper, and then top the salmon again with 2 thin slices of lemon.

7. Close and lock the lid, cooking on "Manual, High Pressure" for 3 minutes.

8. Once done, quick release the pressure.

9. Uncover, and serve immediately.

10. Nutrition Info: Calories 224, Carbs 3g, Fat 13g, Protein 22 g, Potassium (K) 602 mg, Sodium (Na) 581 mg

Mussels and Spaghetti Squash

Servings: 2

Cooking Time: 35 Minutes

Ingredients:

• 1lb cooked, shelled mussels

• 1/2 a spaghetti squash, to fit the Pressure Pot

• 1 cup low sodium fish broth

• 3tbsp crushed garlic

• sea salt to taste

Directions:

1. Mix the mussels with the garlic and salt.

2. Place the mussels inside the squash.

3. Lower the squash into your Pressure Pot.

4. Pour the broth around it.

5. Cook on Stew for 3minutes.

6. Release the pressure naturally.

7. Shred the squash, mixing the "spaghetti" with the mussels.

8. Nutrition Info: Per serving: Calories: 265; Carbs: 7; Sugar: 1 ; Fat: 9 ; Protein: 4; GL: 3

Shrimp with Tomatoes and Feta

Servings: 6

Cooking Time: 12 Minutes

Ingredients:

- 2 tbsp. butter

- 1 lb. frozen shrimp

- 1 tbsp. garlic

- 1½ cups chopped white onion

- 14.5 oz. crushed tomatoes

- 1 tsp. dried oregano

- 1 tsp. sea salt

- ½ tsp. red pepper flakes, or to taste

- To Serve:

- 1 cup crumbled feta cheese

- ½ cup sliced black olives

- ¼ cup fresh parsley

Directions:

1. Select the "Sauté" function on your Pressure Pot and once hot, add the butter.

2. Melt the butter and then add the garlic and red pepper flakes.

3. Next, add in the onions, tomatoes, salt, and oregano.

4. Add the frozen shrimp.

5. Set the Pressure Pot on "Manual, High Pressure" setting for1 minute.

6. Once done, release all the pressure and stir well to combine all the ingredients.

7. Allow to cool and then sprinkle with feta cheese, black olives, and parsley.

8. Serve with buttered French bread, or rice.

9. Nutrition Info: Calories 211, Carbs 6g, Fat 11 g, Protein 1g, Potassium (K) 148 mg, Sodium (Na) 1468 mg

Salmon Bake

Servings: 2

Cooking Time: 15 Minutes

Ingredients:

• 1lb salmon

• 1lb chopped Mediterranean vegetables

• 1 cup low sodium fish broth

• juice of half a lemon

• sea salt as desired

Directions:

1. Mix all the ingredients except the broth in a foil pouch.

2. Place the pouch in the steamer basket your Pressure Pot.

3. Pour the broth into your Pressure Pot.

4. Cook on Steam for 15 minutes.

5. Release the pressure naturally.

6. Nutrition Info: Per serving: Calories: 2; Carbs: 5; Sugar: 1 ; Fat: 12 ; Protein: 36 ; GL: 1

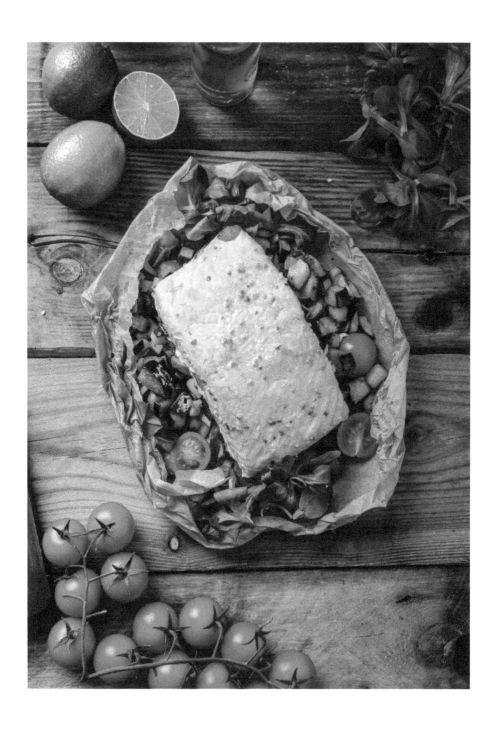

Lemony Mussels

Servings: 4

Cooking Time: 9 Minutes

Ingredients:

• 2 pounds mussels, cleaned and de-bearded

• 1 medium onion, chopped

• ½ teaspoon dried rosemary, crushed

• 1 cup low-sodium chicken broth

• 2 tablespoons fresh lemon juice

• 1 tablespoon olive oil

• 1 garlic clove, minced

• Salt and ground black pepper, as required

Directions:

1. In the Pressure Pot, place oil and press "Sauté". Now add the onion and cook for about 5
 minutes.

2. Stir in the garlic and rosemary and cook for about 1 minute.

3. Press "Cancel" and stir in the broth, lemon juice and black pepper.

4. Arrange the steamer trivet on top of broth mixture in

the Pressure Pot.

5. Close the lid and place the pressure valve to "Seal" position.

6. Place the mussels in a steamer trivet.

7. Press "Manual" and cook under "Low Pressure" for about 2-3 minutes.

8. Press "Cancel" and carefully allow a "Quick" release.

9. Open the lid and transfer the mussels into a serving bowl.

10. Top with the cooking liquid and serve.

11. Nutrition Info: Per serving: Calories: 243, Fats: 8.7g, Carbs: , Sugar: 1.3g, Proteins: 27.9g, Sodium: 700mg

Salmon In Green Sauce

Servings: 4

Cooking Time: 12 Minutes

Ingredients:

• 4 (6-ounce) salmon fillets

• 1 avocado, peeled, pitted and chopped

• ½ cup fresh basil, chopped

• 3 garlic cloves, chopped

• 1 tablespoon fresh lemon zest, grated finely

Directions:

1. Grease a large piece of foil.

2. In a large bowl, add all ingredients except salmon and water and with a fork, mash completely.

3. Place fillets in the center of foil and top with avocado mixture evenly.

4. Fold the foil around fillets to seal them.

5. Arrange a steamer trivet in the Pressure Pot and pour ½ cup of water.

6. Place the foil packet on top of trivet.

7. Close the lid and place the pressure valve to "Seal" position.

8. Press "Manual" and cook under "High Pressure" for about minutes.

9. Meanwhile, preheat the oven to broiler.

10.Press "Cancel" and allow a "Natural" release.

11. Open the lid and transfer the salmon fillets onto a broiler pan.

12. Broil for about 3-4 minutes.

13. Serve warm.

14. Nutrition Info: Per serving: Calories: 333, Fats: 20.3g, Carbs: 5.5g, Sugar: 0.4g, Proteins: 34.2g, Sodium: 79mg

Salmon With Sweet & Spicy Sauce

Servings: 4

Cooking Time: 5 Minutes

Ingredients:

• 4 (5-ounce) salmon fillets

• 2 jalapeño peppers, seeded and chopped finely

• 2 tablespoons fresh parsley, chopped

• 2 tablespoons Yacon syrup 2 tablespoons hot water

• 3 garlic cloves, minced

• 3 tablespoons fresh lime juice

• 2 tablespoons olive oil

• 1 teaspoon ground cumin

• 1 teaspoon paprika Salt and ground black pepper, as required

Directions:

1. Season the salmon fillets with salt and black pepper evenly.

2. Arrange a steamer trivet in the Pressure Pot and pour1 cup of water.

3. Place the salmon fillets on top of trivet.

4. Close the lid and place the pressure valve to "Seal" position.

5. Press "Steam" and just use the default time of minutes.

6. Press "Cancel" and carefully allow a "Quick" release.

7. Meanwhile, for sauce: in a bowl, add the remaining ingredients and mix until well combined.

8. Open the lid and transfer the salmon fillets onto a serving plate.

9. Drizzle with sauce and serve.

10. Nutrition Info: Per serving: Calories: 272, Fats: 16.1g, Carbs: 5g, Sugar: 2.1g, Proteins: 28g, Sodium: 252mg

Rosemary Salmon

Servings: 3

Cooking Time: 15 Minutes

Ingredients:

• 1 tbsp. olive oil

• 1 lb. frozen, wild-caught salmon

• 1 sprig fresh rosemary

• 10 oz. fresh asparagus

• ½ cup halved cherry tomatoes

• 1 tbsp. lemon juice

• 1 tsp. Kosher salt

• Black pepper

Directions:

1. Pour a cup of water into the Pressure Pot and place a wire rack into the pot.

2. Place the fish in a single layer onto the rack, and then add a sprig of rosemary and finally the fresh asparagus.

3. Choose the "Manual, High pressure" setting and adjust the cook time to minutes.

4. Once done, release the pressure and uncover the pot.

5. Remove the lid and transfer all the contents onto a plate, discarding the rosemary.

6. Add the cherry tomatoes, drizzle with olive oil and season with salt and black pepper.

7. Sprinkle with lemon juice and serve.

8. Nutrition Info: Calories 2, Carbs 5g, Fat 14 g, Protein 32 g, Potassium (K) 985 mg, Sodium (Na) 71 mg

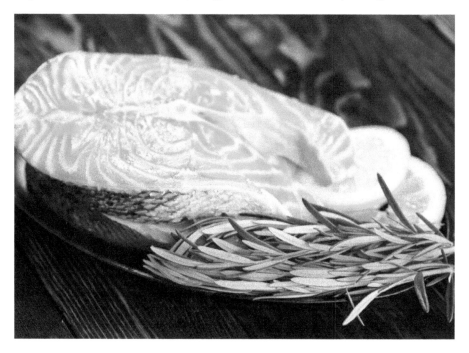

Monk-fish Curry

Servings: 2

Cooking Time: 20 Minutes

Ingredients:

• 0.5lb monkfish

• 1 thinly sliced sweet yellow onion

• 0.5 cup chopped tomato

• 3tbsp strong curry paste

• 1tbsp oil or ghee

Directions:

1. Set the Pressure Pot to sauté and add the onion, oil, and curry paste.

2. When the onion is soft, add the remaining ingredients and seal.

3. Cook on Stew for 20 minutes.

4. Release the pressure naturally.

5. Nutrition Info: Per serving: Calories: 270; Carbs: 1; Sugar: 6; Fat: 11; Protein: 4; GL: 12

Coconut Shrimp Curry

Servings: 4

Cooking Time: 15 Minutes

Ingredients:

- 1 tbsp. vegetable oil
- 1 lb. frozen shrimp
- 1 cup chopped white onion
- ½ tbsp. minced ginger
- ½ tbsp. minced garlic
- 1 tsp. mustard seeds
- 1 green chili pepper
- 1 cup chopped tomato
- ¼ can coconut milk
- 1 tbsp. lime juice
- ¼ cup cilantro
- For the Spice mix:
- 1 tsp. coriander powder
- ½ tsp. cayenne or red chili powder
- ½ tsp. ground turmeric
- ½ tsp. garam masala
- ½ tsp. sea salt

Directions:

1. Select the "Sauté" function on the Pressure Pot and allow it to heat up.

2. Add the oil and mustard seeds and sizzle them until they begin to pop.

3. Add the onions, ginger, garlic and green chili.

4. Sauté for 5 minutes until the onions are a light golden brown and the garlic and ginger aromatic.

5. Add the tomato and all the spices. Mix and sauté for 2-3 minutes.

6. Now, add the coconut milk and shrimp. Stir and select the "Cancel" button. Close the lid with steam release vent in the "Sealing" position.

7. Cook on the "Manual, Low Pressure" setting for 3 minutes.

8. Once done, quick release the pressure manually.

9. Stir in the lime and garnish with cilantro.

10. Enjoy and serve with rice.

11. Nutrition Info: Calories 226, Carbs 8g, Fat 10 g, Protein 24 g, Potassium (K) 289 mg, Sodium (Na) 1222 mg

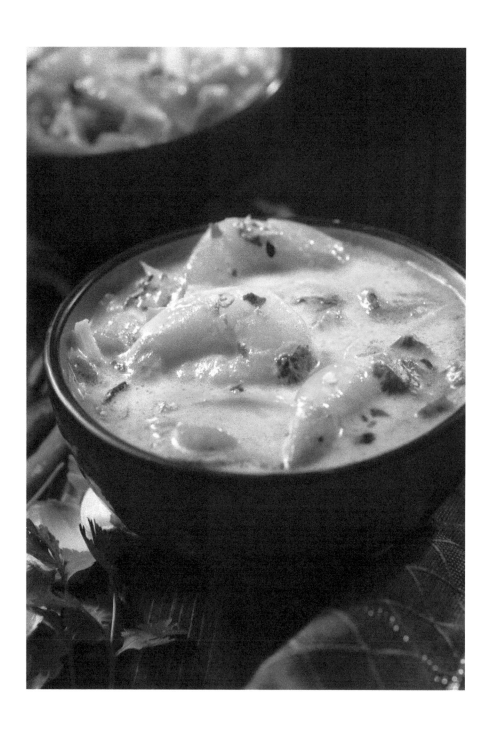

Sweet & Sour Tuna

Servings: 4

Cooking Time: 9 Minutes

Ingredients:

• 4 (6-ounce) tuna steaks, pat dried

• ½ cup low-sodium chicken broth

• 2 tablespoon Yacon syrup

• 2 tablespoon balsamic vinegar

• 2 tablespoons kaffir lime leaves, minced

• 1 (½-inch) piece fresh ginger, minced

• Ground black pepper, as required

Directions:

1. In the pot of Pressure Pot, place all the ingredients and mix well.

2. Add the tuna steaks and mix with broth mixture.

3. Secure the lid and place the pressure valve to "Seal" position

4. Press "Manual" and cook under "High Pressure" for about 6 minutes.

5. Press "Cancel" and carefully allow a "Quick" release.

6. Open the lid and with a slotted spoon, transfer the

tuna steaks onto a plate.

7. Press "Sauté" and cook for about 2-3 minutes or until sauce becomes slightly thick.

8. Press "Cancel" and pour the sauce over tuna steaks.

9. Serve immediately.

10. Nutrition Info: Per serving: Calories: 329, Fats: 7g, Carbs: 3.3g, Sugar: 1.8g, Proteins: 5.1g, Sodium: 97mg

Tuna And Cheddar

Servings: 2

Cooking Time: 35 Minutes

Ingredients:

• 3 small cans tuna

• 1lb finely chopped vegetables

• 1 cup low sodium vegetable broth

• 0.5 cup shredded cheddar

Directions:

1. Mix all the ingredients in your Pressure Pot.

2. Cook on Stew for 35 minutes.

3. Release the pressure naturally.

4. Nutrition Info: Per serving: Calories: 320; Carbs: 8; Sugar: 2 ; Fat: 11 ; Protein: 37 ; GL: 4

Cod In Parsley Sauce

Servings: 2

Cooking Time: 5 Minutes

Ingredients:

• 1lb boneless, skinless cod fillets

• 0.5lb green peas

• 1 cup white sauce

• juice of a lemon

• 2tbsp dry parsley

Directions:

1. Mix all the ingredients in your Pressure Pot.

2. Cook on Stew for 35 minutes.

3. Release the pressure naturally.

4. Nutrition Info: Per serving: Calories: 330; Carbs: 8 ; Sugar: 1 ; Fat: 19 ; Protein: ; GL: 3

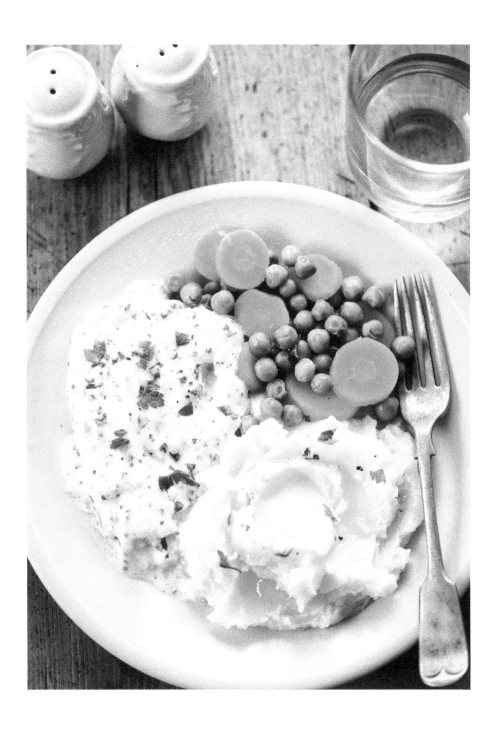

Beer-braised Chicken with Grape-apple Slaw

Servings: 8

Cooking Time: 20 Minutes

Ingredients:

• For the chicken

• 1 cup brown ale

• 1 teaspoon white wheat flour

• 2 bone-in, skin-on chicken breasts (about 2 pounds)

• Kosher salt

• Freshly ground black pepper

• 1 tablespoon coarse-grain mustard

• For the slaw

• ¼ cup cider vinegar

• 2 tablespoons extra-virgin olive oil

• 1 tablespoon honey

• 1 tablespoon coarse-grain mustard

• Kosher salt

• Freshly ground black pepper

• ¼ head purple or red cabbage, thinly sliced

• 2 cups seedless green grapes, halved

- 1 medium apple, cut into matchstick-size slices (I like Gala)

Directions:

1. To make the chicken

2. In a cup measuring cup or small bowl, whisk together the ale and flour. Pour into the electric pressure cooker.

3. Sprinkle the chicken breasts with salt and pepper. Place them in the electric pressure cooker, meat-side down.

4. Close and lock the lid of the pressure cooker. Set the valve to sealing.

5. Cook on high pressure for 20 minutes. While the chicken is cooking, make the slaw.

6. When the cooking is complete, hit Cancel. Allow the pressure to release naturally for 5

minutes, then quick release any remaining pressure.

7. Once the pin drops, unlock and remove the lid.

8. Using tongs, remove the chicken breasts to a cutting board. Hit Sauté/More and bring the liquid in the pot to a boil, scraping up any brown bits on the bottom of

the pot. Cook, stirring occasionally, for about 5 minutes or until the sauce has reduced in volume by about a third. Hit Cancel and whisk in the mustard.

9. When the chicken is cool enough to handle, remove the skin, shred the meat, and return it to the pot. Let the chicken soak in the sauce for at least 5 minutes.

10. Serve the chicken topped with the slaw.

11. To make the slaw

12. In a small jar with a screw-top lid, combine the vinegar, olive oil, honey, and mustard. Shake well, then season with salt and pepper, and shake again.

13. In a large bowl, toss together the cabbage, grapes, and apple. Add the dressing and mix well. Let the mixture sit at room temperature while the chicken cooks.

14. Nutrition Info: Per serving(½ CUP CHICKEN, PLUS ½ CUP SLAW): Calories: 203; Total Fat: 9g; Protein: 13g; Carbohydrates: 16g; Sugars: 12g; Fiber: 2g; Sodium: 80mg

Sweet & Tangy Pulled Chicken

Servings: 3

Cooking Time: 11 Minutes

Ingredients:

• 2 (6-ounce) boneless, skinless chicken breasts, halved lengthwise

• ¼ cup yacon syrup

• ½ of yellow onion, chopped roughly

• ½ tablespoon arrowroot starch

• 1 tablespoon water

• 1 tablespoon olive oil

• ¼ cup fresh lemon juice

• 1 tablespoon garlic, minced

• 1 teaspoon fresh ginger, minced

• 1 teaspoon red pepper flakes, crushed

• Salt and freshly ground black pepper, required

Directions:

1. For sauce: in a bowl, add all ingredients except chicken breasts, arrowroot starch and water and beat until well combined.

2. In the bottom of Pressure Pot, place the chicken

breast halves and top with the sauce.

3. Close the lid and place the pressure valve to "Seal" position.

4. Press "Manual" and cook under "High Pressure" for about 5 minutes.

5. Press "Cancel" and carefully allow a "Quick" release.

6. Open the lid and with tongs, transfer the chicken breast halves into a bowl.

7. With 2 forks, shred chicken.

8. In a bowl, dissolve the arrowroot starch into water.

9. Now, press "Sauté" and add arrowroot starch mixture, stirring continuously.

10. Cook for about 2 minutes or until desired thickness of sauce, stirring occasionally.

11. Add the shredded chicken and stir to combine.

12.Press "Cancel" and serve hot.

13. Nutrition Info: Per serving: Calories: 314, Fats: 4g, Carbs: 13g, Sugar: 6g, Proteins: 33.5g, Sodium: 162mg

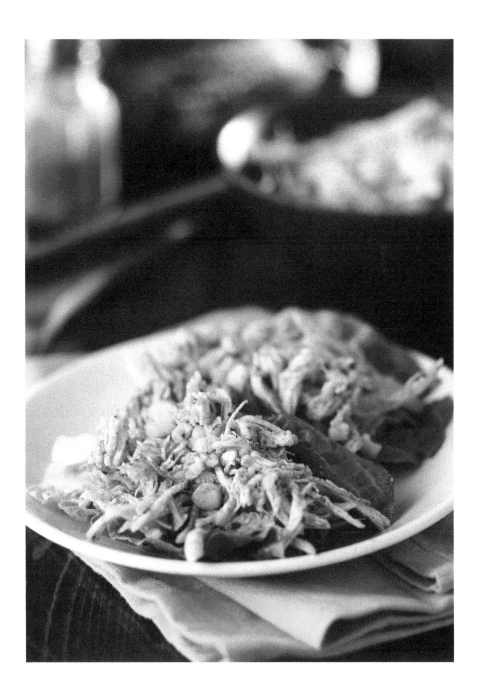

Chicken Coconut Curry

Servings: 2

Cooking Time: 20 Minutes

Ingredients:

• 0.5lb chopped cooked chicken breast

• 1 thinly sliced onion

• 1 cup coconut milk

• 3tbsp curry paste

• 1tbsp oil or ghee

Directions:

1. Set the Pressure Pot to sauté and add the onion, oil, and curry paste.

2. When the onion is soft, add the remaining ingredients and seal.

3. Cook on Stew for 20 minutes.

4. Release the pressure naturally.

5. Nutrition Info: Per serving: Calories: 4; Carbs: 27; Sugar: 16 ; Fat: 25 ; Protein: 43 ; GL: 21

Lemon Cilantro Chicken

Servings: 2

Cooking Time: 35 Minutes

Ingredients:

• 1lb diced chicken breast

• 1lb chopped vegetables

• 1 cup chicken broth

• juice of half a lemon

• 2tbsp dry cilantro

Directions:

1. Mix all the ingredients in your Pressure Pot.

2. Cook on Stew for 35 minutes.

3. Release the pressure naturally.

4. Nutrition Info: Per serving: Calories: 280; Carbs:

Sugar: 0 ; Fat: 12 ; Protein: 45 ; GL: 1

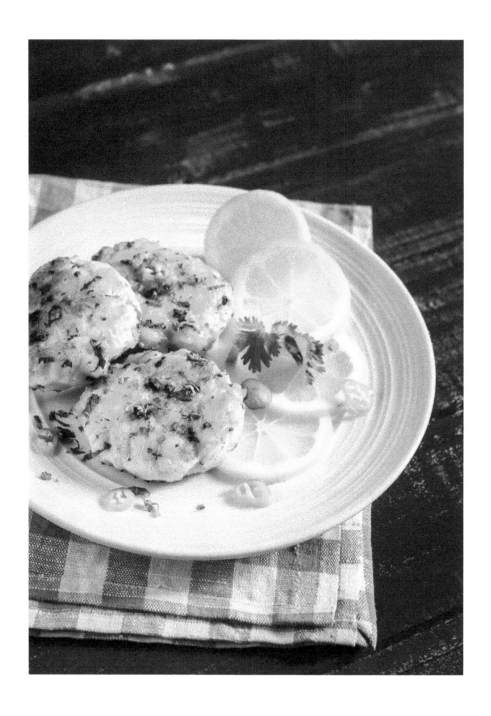

Pressure Pot Chicken Breast

Servings: 8

Cooking Time: 20 Minutes

Ingredients:

• 3 lbs. boneless and skinless chicken breasts

• 1 cup water

• 2 tsp. garlic powder

• Black pepper

• 1 tsp. salt

Directions:

1. Pour in water into the Pressure Pot and place a trivet with handles inside.

2. Place the chicken breasts into the Pressure Pot, arranging them in a single layer.

3. If using frozen chicken make sure each breast is separated, and not touching each other.

4. Season with garlic powder, black pepper, and salt, toss well to mix using tongs or your hands.

5. Close and seal the lid, setting the pressure release vent to "Sealing" and choose the "Manual, High Pressure" setting.

6. Cook for 20 minutes if using fresh chicken or 25 minutes if using frozen chicken breasts.

7. The Pressure Pot will take 10 minutes to come to pressure, so factor this time in your cooking.

8. After the cook cycle is done, the Pressure Pot will beep, and will need about 20 minutes to come down to pressure. This is known as a Natural Pressure Release and should take about 10-15 minutes.

9. A quick release will not work for this recipe, as it makes the meat tough.

10. Carefully open the lid and use the chicken breasts for meal prep, casseroles, salads etc.

11. Shred or cube the chicken and save the stock for other recipes like soup.

12. Nutrition Info: Calories 204, Carbs 0 g, Fat 4.5 g, Protein 38.3 g, Potassium (K) 496 mg, Sodium (Na) 294.5 mg

Buffalo Pulled Chicken

Servings: 6

Cooking Time: 29 Minutes

Ingredients:

• 4 (6-ounce) boneless, skinless chicken breasts

• 1 cup low-sodium chicken broth

• ½ cup hot sauce

Directions:

1. In the pot of Pressure Pot, place chicken breasts and broth.

2. Close the lid and place the pressure valve to "Seal" position.

3. Press "Manual" and cook under "High Pressure" for about 26 minutes.

4. Press "Cancel" and carefully allow a "Quick" release.

5. Open the lid and transfer the chicken breasts onto a platter.

6. With 2 forks, shred the chicken breasts.

7. Remove the broth from pot, leaving about ½ cup inside.

8. Press "Sauté" and stir in shredded chicken and hot

sauce.

9. Cook for about 2-3 minutes, stirring continuously.

10.Press "Cancel" and serve hot.

11. Nutrition Info: Per serving: Calories: 220, Fats: 8.5g, Carbs: 0.5g, Sugar: 0.2g, Proteins: 33.2g, Sodium: 617mg

Balsamic Turkey Breast

Servings: 2

Cooking Time: 35 Minutes

Ingredients:

- 1lb diced turkey breast

- 1lb chopped vegetables

- 1 cup chicken soup

- 2tbsp balsamic reduction

Directions:

1. Mix all the ingredients in your Pressure Pot.

2. Cook on Stew for 35 minutes.

3. Release the pressure naturally.

4. Nutrition Info: Per serving: Calories: 295; Carbs: 5; Sugar: 2; Fat: 1; Protein: 46 ; GL: 2

Turkey Chili

Servings: 6

Cooking Time: 40 Minutes

Ingredients:

- 1 1/2 cup frozen corn
- 15-ounce cooked black beans
- 1-pound ground turkey
- 14.5-ounce diced tomatoes
- 1 teaspoon garlic powder
- ¾ teaspoon salt
- 2 tablespoons red chili powder
- 1 tablespoon cumin
- 1 ½ teaspoon smoked paprika
- 1 teaspoon dried basil
- 1 teaspoon oregano
- 1 cup water

Directions:

1. Plugin Pressure Pot, insert the inner pot, add turkey, and then add remaining ingredients.

2. Shut the Pressure Pot with its lid, turn the pressure knob to seal the pot, then press the „manual" button,

then press the „timer" to set the cooking time to minutes and cook at high pressure, Pressure Pot will take 5 minutes or more for building its inner pressure.

3. When the timer beeps, press „cancel" button and do quick pressure release until pressure nob drops down.

4. Open the Pressure Pot, stir the chili and evenly divide between serving bowls.

5. Serve straight away.

6. Nutrition Info: Calories: 220 Cal, Carbs: 22 g, Fat: 7 g, Protein: 20 g, Fiber: 5 g.

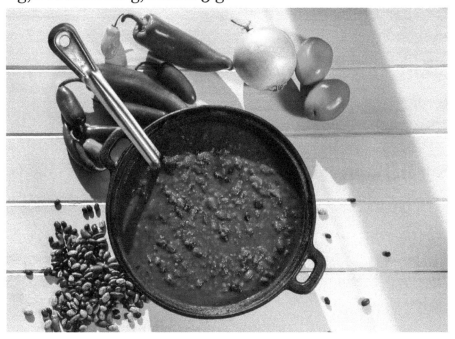

Spicy Mixed Greens

Servings: 6

Cooking Time: 9 Minutes

Ingredients:

• 2 medium onions, chopped

• 1 pound mustard leaves, rinsed

• 1 pound fresh spinach, rinsed

• 2 tablespoons olive oil

• 4 garlic cloves, minced

• 1 (2-inch) piece fresh ginger, minced

• 1 teaspoon ground cumin

• 1 teaspoon ground coriander ½ teaspoon red chili powder

• ½ teaspoon ground turmeric

• Salt and ground black pepper, as required

Directions:

1. In the Pressure Pot, place oil and press "Sauté". Now add the onion, garlic, ginger, and spices and cook for about 2-3 minutes.

2. Add the greens and cook for about minutes.

3. Press "Cancel" and stir well.

4. Close the lid and place the pressure valve to "Seal" position.

5. Press "Manual" and cook under "High Pressure" for about 4 minutes.

6. Press "Cancel" and allow a "Natural" release.

7. Open the lid and with an immersion blender, puree the mixture until smooth.

8. Serve immediately.

9. Nutrition Info: Per serving: Calories: , Fats: 5.3g, Carbs: 11g, Sugar: 3.2g, Proteins: 4.8g, Sodium: 110mg

Cilantro Lime Chicken

Servings: 6

Cooking Time: 15 Minutes

Ingredients:

• 2 lbs. boneless and skinless chicken breasts

• 1 chopped jalapeño

• 24 oz. no-sugar salsa

• 14 oz. low-sodium black beans

• 1 packet low-sodium taco seasoning

• ¼ cup water or low-sodium chicken stock

• Juice and zest of 1 lime

 To Garnish:

• Chopped cilantro

Directions:

1. Take a 6-quart or larger Pressure Pot and add to it all the ingredients for the chicken, except the fresh cilantro.

 2. Close and seal the lid, making sure the pressure valve is set to "Sealing", and then cook on "Manual, High Pressure" for 15 minutes.

 3. Once the cook cycle is up, allow for a natural

pressure release for 10 minutes, followed by a quick release of any remaining pressure.

4. Uncover, and using two forks, shred the chicken breast.

5. Add the chopped cilantro and then stir everything well to incorporate all the ingredients.

6. Serve, top with your favorite toppings, and enjoy!

7. Nutrition Info: Calories 2, Carbs 27g, Fat 4 g, Protein 33 g, Potassium (K) 188.5 mg, Sodium (Na) 102.5 mg

Spicy Black Beans

Servings: 4

Cooking Time: 35 Minutes

Ingredients:

• 1 cup black beans, soaked overnight and drained

• 1 medium onion, chopped

• 2 cups water

• 1 tablespoon olive oil

• 1 teaspoon cumin seeds

• 1 tablespoon garlic paste

• 1 tablespoon ginger paste

• 2 teaspoons ground coriander

• 1 teaspoon red chili powder

• ½ teaspoon ground turmeric

• Salt, as required

• 1 teaspoon fresh lemon juice

Directions:

1. In the Pressure Pot, place oil and press "Sauté". Now add the cumin seeds and cook for about 30 seconds.

2. Add the onion, ginger, garlic and spices and cook for about 3-4 minutes.

3. Press "Cancel" and stir in the chickpeas and water.

4. Close the lid and place the pressure valve to "Seal" position.

5. Press "Beans/Chili" and just use the default time of 30 minutes.

6. Press "Cancel" and allow a "Natural" release.

7. Open the lid and stir in lemon juice.

8. Serve hot.

9. Nutrition Info: Per serving: Calories: 137, Fats: 4.6g, Carbs: 13g, Sugar: 2.1g, Proteins: 6g, Sodium: 56mg

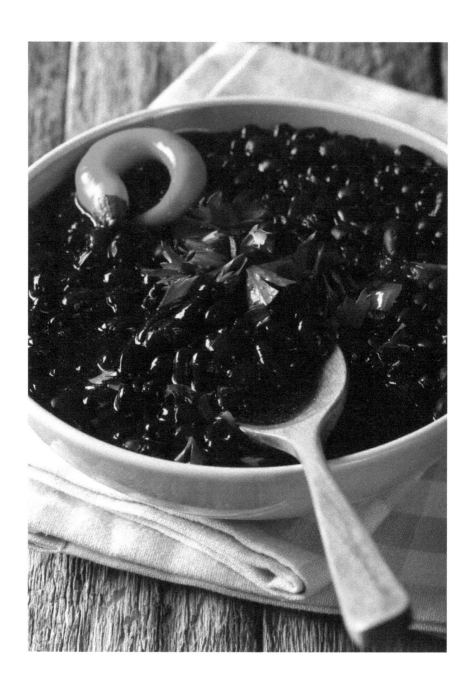

Herbed Chicken Breasts

Servings: 4

Cooking Time: 13 Minutes

Ingredients:

• 4 (4-ounce) boneless, skinless chicken breasts

• ½ teaspoon dried oregano, crushed

• ½ teaspoon dried basil, crushed

• 1 teaspoon garlic powder

• Ground black pepper, as required

• 1 tablespoon olive oil

Directions:

1. Season the chicken with garlic powder and black pepper generously.

2. In the Pressure Pot, place oil and press "Sauté". Now add the chicken breasts and cook for about 3-4 minutes per side.

3. Press "Cancel" and transfer the chicken breasts onto a plate.

4. Arrange a steamer trivet in the Pressure Pot and pour 1¼ cups water.

5. Arrange the chicken breasts on top of trivet.

6. Close the lid and place the pressure valve to "Seal" position.

7. Press "Manual" and cook under "High Pressure" for about 5 minutes.

8. Press "Cancel" and carefully allow a "Quick" release.

9. Open the lid and serve hot.

10. Nutrition Info: Per serving: Calories: 248, Fats: 11.9g, Carbs: 0.7g, Sugar: 0.2g, Proteins: 33g, Sodium: 98mg.

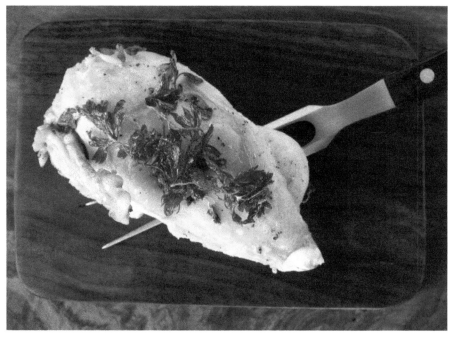

Chicken With Cauliflower

Servings: 6

Cooking Time: 22 Minutes

Ingredients:

• 1½ pounds boneless, skinless chicken thighs, cubed

• ½ onion, chopped

• 2 cups tomatoes, crushed finely

• 2½ cups cauliflower florets

• ¾ cup water

• ½ tablespoon olive oil

• 1 teaspoon fresh ginger root, minced

• 3 garlic cloves, minced

• 1 teaspoon ground cumin

• 1 teaspoon ground coriander

• ½ teaspoon ground turmeric

• ½ teaspoon cayenne pepper

• Salt, as required

Directions:

1. In the Pressure Pot, place oil and press "Sauté". Now add the onion, ginger, garlic and spices and cook for about 2-3 minutes.

2. Add the tomatoes and stir to combine.

3. Press "Cancel" and stir in the chicken and water.

4. Close the lid and place the pressure valve to "Seal" position.

5. Press "Manual" and cook under "High Pressure" for about 1minutes.

6. Press "Cancel" and carefully allow a "Quick" release.

7. Open the lid and stir in the cauliflower and crushed tomatoes.

8. Press "Manual" and cook under "High Pressure" for about 2 minutes.

9. Press "Cancel" and carefully allow a "Quick" release.

10. Open the lid and serve hot.

11. Nutrition Info: Per serving: Calories: 255, Fats: 9.9g, Carbs: 6.3g, Sugar: 3g, Proteins: 34.5g, Sodium: 142mg

Half Roast Chicken

Servings: 2

Cooking Time: 35 Minutes

Ingredients:

• half a chicken

• 2tbsp mixed herbs

• 2tbsp rub

• 1 cup low sodium broth

Directions:

1. Mix all the herbs, rub, and a little broth and rub it into the chicken.

2. Pour the broth in your Pressure Pot and lower the chicken, bones down.

3. Cook on Stew for minutes.

4. Release the pressure naturally.

5. Nutrition Info: Per serving: Calories: 300; Carbs: 6; Sugar: 1 ; Fat: 9 ; Protein: 43 ; GL: 2

Chicken In Spicy Yogurt Sauce

Servings: 6

Cooking Time: 20 Minutes

Ingredients:

• 2 pounds boneless, skinless chicken breasts, cubed

• ½ cup onion, sliced thinly

• 2 cups tomatoes, chopped

• ½ cup low-sodium chicken broth

• ¼ cup fat-free plain Greek yogurt, whipped

• 2 tablespoons olive oil

• 2 tablespoons curry powder

• 1 tablespoon fresh ginger, minced

• 1 tablespoon garlic, minced garlic

• Ground black pepper, as required

Directions:

1. In the Pressure Pot, place oil and press "Sauté". Now add the chicken pieces and cook for about 3-4 minutes.

2. With a slotted spoon, transfer the chicken into a bowl.

3. In the pot, add the onion, ginger, garlic and curry powder and cook for about 2-minutes.

4. Press "Cancel" and stir in the tomatoes, yogurt, broth and black pepper.

5. Close the lid and place the pressure valve to "Seal" position.

6. Press "Manual" and cook under "High Pressure" for about 12 minutes.

7. Press "Cancel" and carefully allow a "Quick" release.

8. Open the lid and stir in cooked chicken.

9. Close the lid and place the pressure valve to "Seal" position.

10.Press "Manual" and cook under "High Pressure" for about 3 minutes.

11.Press "Cancel" and allow a "Natural" release.

12. Open the lid and serve hot.

13. Nutrition Info: Per serving: Calories: 359, Fats: 16.3g, Carbs: 5.5g, Sugar: 2.5g, Proteins: 45.9g, Sodium: 145mg

Chicken Tacos

Servings: 10

Cooking Time: 25 Minutes

Ingredients:

• 4 pounds chicken breast

• 1/2 of a medium head of lettuce, shredded

• 3 medium avocados, pitted and flesh chopped

• 1 medium white onion, peeled and chopped

• 3 limes, juiced

• 2 jalapeno peppers, deseeded and diced

• 1 teaspoon onion powder

• 1 teaspoon garlic powder

• 1 ¾ teaspoon salt

• 1 teaspoon ground black pepper

• 1 ½ teaspoon red chili powder

• 1 ½ teaspoon ground cumin

• 2 tablespoons olive oil

Directions:

1. Place lettuce, avocado, onion, and pepper in a large bowl, drizzle with lime juice and toss until coated, chill vegetables in the refrigerator for 30 minutes.

2. Meanwhile, plug-in Pressure Pot, insert the inner pot, pour in water, then insert trivet stand and place chicken on it.

3. Shut the Pressure Pot with its lid, turn the pressure knob to seal the pot, press the „manual" button, then press the „timer" to set the cooking time to 10 minutes and cook at high pressure, Pressure Pot will take 5 minutes or more for building its inner pressure.

4. When the timer beeps, press „cancel" button and do quick pressure release until pressure nob drops down.

5. Open the Pressure Pot, transfer chicken breasts to a cutting board, cool for minutes, then shred with two forks.

6. Place shredded chicken in a bowl and season with salt, black pepper, red chili, and cumin until evenly coated.

7. Drain the Pressure Pot, wipe clean the inner pot, then press the „sauté/simmer" button, grease with oil and when hot, add seasoned chicken in a single layer and cook for 3 to 5 minutes or until chicken is nicely golden brown and slightly crispy.

8. Serve chicken in tortillas, topped with prepared vegetables.

9. Nutrition Info: Calories: 164.4 Cal, Carbs: 8.3 g, Fat: 11.1 g, Protein: 10.1 g, Fiber: 4.8 g.

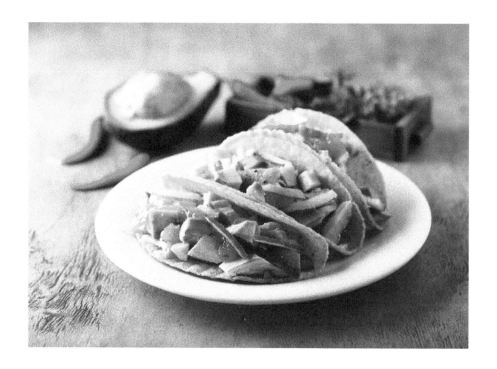

Lemon Chicken with Garlic

Servings: 8

Cooking Time: 20 Minutes

Ingredients:

• 2 tbsps. olive oil

• 3 tbsps. butter

• 8 skinless, boneless chicken thighs

• ½ chopped white onion

• 4 minced garlic cloves

• ⅓ cup low-sodium chicken broth

• 2 tbsps. heavy cream

• 4 tsps. Italian seasoning

• ½ tsp. smoked paprika

• ½ tsp. garlic powder

• ½ tsp. red chili flakes optional or to taste

• Zest of ½ a lemon

• Juice of 1 lemon

• Coarse sea salt

• Black pepper

• To Garnish:

- Lemon slices
- Chopped parsley

Directions:

1. Season the skin and cavity of the chicken with paprika, garlic powder, sea salt, black pepper, garlic powder, and chili flakes.

2. Select the "Sauté" function on Normal on your Pressure Pot.

3. Add olive oil to the inner pot of a large 6-quart Pressure Pot and allow it to get hot.

4. Place the seasoned chicken into the Pressure Pot and cook for 2-3 minutes per side, until golden brown.

5. Once the chicken is light and golden brown, remove the chicken from Pressure Pot and set it aside.

6. Melt the butter, and stir in the chopped onions and minced garlic.

7. Deglaze the pot with lemon juice, and cook for 1 minute.

8. Now add the Italian seasoning, chicken broth, and lemon zest.

9. Return the chicken into the Pressure Pot, and then

close and seal the lid, turning the steam release valve to "Sealing."

10. Select the "Manual, High Pressure" setting on older models or the "Pressure Cook" setting on newer models, and cook for 7 minutes. Note that the Pressure Pot will take 5-minutes to come up to pressure.

11. Once done, quick release the pressure after 2 minutes, and then uncover the pot.

12. Remove the chicken using tongs and then it set aside.

13. Take the heavy cream and stir it into the Pressure Pot.

14. You may also add a cornstarch, arrowroot starch slurry, or xanthan gum, by mixing ½ a teaspoon cornstarch or arrowroot starch) mixed with 1 teaspoon of cold water.

15. Press the "Off" button, turning the Pressure Pot to the "Sauté" function.

16. Allow the sauce to thicken, and then turn off the pot and add the chicken back into the pot.

17. Spoon the cooking juices all over the chicken and garnish with chopped parsley.

18. Serve with creamed mashed cauliflower, and garnish with lemon slices, if desired.

19. Nutrition Info Calories 282, Carbs 2g, Fat 15 g, Protein 14 g, Potassium (K) 317.0 mg, Sodium (Na) 416 mg

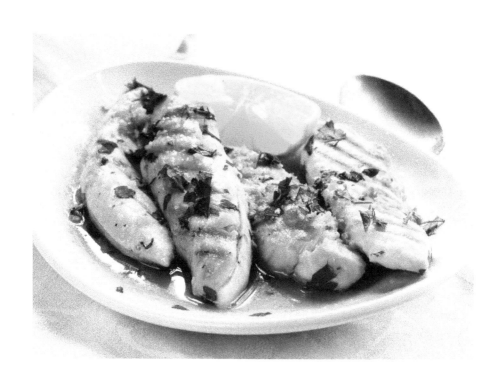

Buffalo Chicken Chili

Servings: 8

Cooking Time: 30 Minutes

Ingredients:

- 2 lbs. skinless and boneless chicken breasts
- 1 chopped white onion
- 5 minced garlic cloves
- 3 chopped carrots
- 3 chopped celery stalks
- 28 oz. diced tomatoes
- 15 oz. low-sodium beans
- ¼ cup Frank"s red hot sauce
- 2 tbsps. maple syrup or honey
- 1 tbsp. chili powder
- 1 tbsp. ground cuminutes
- 1 tbsp. smoked paprika
- ½ tsp. salt
- ½ crumbled blue cheese

Directions:

1. In your Pressure Pot, add all the ingredients, staring with the garlic, onion, carrots, celery, beans, maple

syrup, ground cumin, chili powder, smoked paprika, salt, chicken, hot sauce and finish with the canned diced tomatoes. Do not stir the mixture.

2. Close and seal the lid and set the steam release vent to "Sealing" and choose to cook on the "Manual, High Pressure" setting for 30 minutes.

3. Once cooked, release the pressure, by performing a quick pressure release. Turn the steam release valve to the "Venting" position until the dial completely drops down.

4. Remove the chicken breasts, shred, and return to the Pressure Pot.

5. Add blue cheese, stir and rest for a few minutes.

6. Serve hot, garnished with green onion, cilantro, and lime.

7. Nutrition Info: Calories 313, Carbs 29.2g, Fat 6 g, Protein 35.1 g, Potassium (K) 6.5 mg, Sodium (Na) 728.2 mg

Firecracker Chicken Meatballs

Servings:

Cooking Time: 6 Minutes

Ingredients:

- For the sauce
- ½ cup hot sauce (such as Frank's RedHot)
- 2 tablespoons honey
- 2 tablespoons low-sodium soy sauce or tamari
- For the meatballs
- 1 pound ground chicken or turkey
- 1 cup Panko breadcrumbs (whole wheat, if possible)
- 1 large egg, slightly beaten
- 1½ teaspoons garlic pepper
- 1 teaspoon onion powder
- ¼ teaspoon kosher salt
- 2 tablespoons avocado oil, divided

Directions:

1. To make the sauce

2. In a 1-cup measuring cup, whisk together the hot sauce, honey, and soy sauce.

3. To make the meatballs

4. In a large bowl, combine the chicken, Panko, egg, garlic pepper, onion powder, and salt. Mix gently with your hands until just combined. (Do not overmix or your meatballs will be tough.)

5. Pinch off about a tablespoon of the meat mixture and roll it into a ball. (A 1½-inch cookie scoop makes the job easy.) Repeat with the remaining meat. You should end up with about 30 (1½-inch) meatballs.

6. Set the electric pressure cooker to the Sauté/More setting. When the pot is hot, pour in 1 tablespoon of avocado oil.

7. Add half of the meatballs around the edge of the pot and brown them for 3 to 5 minutes. (The oil tends to pool towards the outside of the pot, so the meatballs will get browner if you put them there. Leaving space in the middle of the pot will also make it easier to turn the meatballs.) Flip the meatballs over and brown the other side for 3 to 5 minutes. Transfer to a paper towel–lined plate and repeat with the remaining 1 tablespoon of avocado oil and meatballs. Hit Cancel.

8. Return the meatballs to the pot and pour in the

sauce mixture. Stir to coat all sides of the meatballs with sauce, then arrange them in a single layer.

9. Close and lock the lid of the pressure cooker. Set the valve to sealing.

10. Cook on high pressure for 6 minutes.

11. When the cooking is complete, hit Cancel. Allow the pressure to release naturally for 10 minutes, then quick release any remaining pressure.

12. Once the pin drops, unlock and remove the lid. Stir to evenly distribute the sauce.

13. Serve with toothpicks as an appetizer or as a main dish.

14. Nutrition Info: Per serving(5 MEATBALLS): Calories: 244; Total Fat: 12g; Protein: 18g; Carbohydrates: 17g; Sugars: 7g; Fiber: 2g; Sodium: 989mg

Chicken Stuffed Potatoes

Servings: 4

Cooking Time: 30 Minutes

Ingredients:

• 6-ounce chicken sausage links

• 4 medium potatoes, each about 8-ounce

• 1 medium zucchini, chopped

• 1 cup chopped green onion

• 1/8 teaspoon salt

• ¼ teaspoon ground black pepper

• ½ teaspoon dried oregano

• 1 teaspoon hot sauce

• 2 tablespoons olive oil, divided

• 2 cups water

• 2 tablespoons crumbled blue cheese, reduced fat

Directions:

1. Plugin Pressure Pot, insert the inner pot, press sauté/simmer button, add tablespoon oil and when hot, add chicken sausage and cook for 3 minutes or until edges are nicely golden brown.

2. Add zucchini and ¾ cup green onion, sprinkle with oregano, pour in 1/3 cup water and cook for 3 minutes or until tender crisp.

3. Then transfer vegetables from the Pressure Pot to a bowl, drizzle with remaining oil and hot sauce, toss until mixed and keep warm by covering the bowl.

4. Press the cancel button, pour in the remaining water, then insert steamer basket and place potatoes on it.

5. Shut the Pressure Pot with its lid, turn the pressure knob to seal the pot, press the „manual" button, then press the „timer" to set the cooking time to 18 minutes and cook at high pressure, Pressure Pot will take minutes or more for building its inner pressure.

6. When the timer beeps, press „cancel" button and do quick pressure release until pressure nob drops down.

7. Open the Pressure Pot, transfer potatoes to a plate, let cool for 5 minutes, then cut each potato in half.

8. Use fork to fluff potatoes, then season with salt and black pepper and evenly top with prepared sausage and zucchini mixture.

9. Sprinkle remaining green onions and cheese on loaded potatoes and serve straight away.

10. Nutrition Info: Calories: 350 Cal, Carbs: 45 g, Fat: 12 g, Protein: 16 g, Fiber: 6 g.

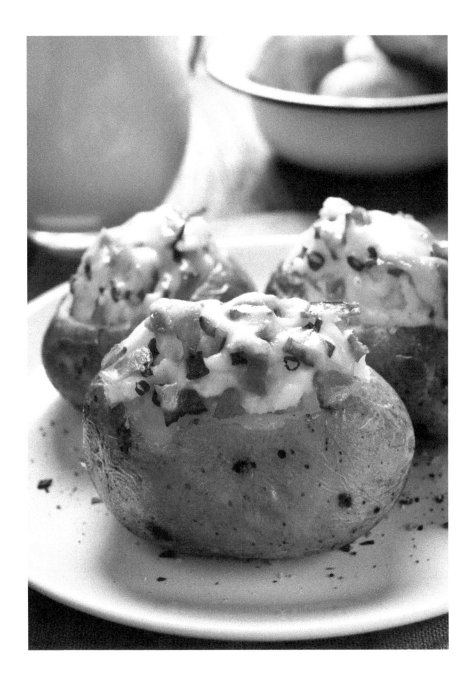

Thai Green Turkey Curry

Servings: 2

Cooking Time: 20 Minutes

Ingredients:

• 0.5lb chopped cooked turkey

• 0.5 cup minced scallions and greens

• 0.5 cup chopped tomato

• 3tbsp Thai green curry paste

• 1tbsp oil or ghee

Directions:

1. Set the Pressure Pot to sauté and add the oil and curry paste.

2. When mixed, add the remaining ingredients and seal.

3. Cook on Stew for 20 minutes.

4. Release the pressure naturally.

5. Nutrition Info: Per serving: Calories: 3; Carbs: 16; Sugar: 5 ; Fat: 15 ; Protein: 43 ; GL: 12

Chicken Salsa Verde with Pumpkin

Servings: 4

Cooking Time: 5 Minutes

Ingredients:

• 2 tablespoons avocado oil

• 1 small onion, chopped

• ½ tablespoon dried oregano

• 3 garlic cloves, finely minced

• 1 cup Chicken Bone Broth or Vegetable Broth

• ¾ cup canned pumpkin purée

• 1 cup Roasted Tomatillo Salsa or salsa verde

• 2 cups shredded cooked chicken breast

• Thinly sliced jalapeño chiles, for garnish (optional)

• Chopped fresh cilantro, for garnish (optional)

Directions:

1. Set the electric pressure cooker to the Sauté setting. When the pot is hot, pour in the avocado oil.

2. Sauté the onion for 3 to 5 minutes or until it begins to soften. Hit Cancel.

3. Stir in the oregano, garlic, broth, pumpkin, salsa, and chicken.

4. Close and lock the lid of the pressure cooker. Set the valve to sealing.

5. Cook on high pressure for minutes.

6. When the cooking is complete, hit Cancel and quick release the pressure.

7. Once the pin drops, unlock and remove the lid.

8. Spoon into serving bowls and garnish with jalapeños and cilantro (if using).

9. Nutrition Info: Per serving(1 CUP): Calories: 238; Total Fat: 10g; Protein: 23g; Carbohydrates: 13g; Sugars: 5g; Fiber: 4g; Sodium: 407mg

Teriyaki Chicken

Servings: 4

Cooking Time: 15 Minutes

Ingredients:

• 3 tablespoons low-sodium gluten-free tamari or soy sauce

• ¼ cup canned crushed pineapple

• 2 tablespoons dark brown sugar

• 2 tablespoons minced garlic

• 1 tablespoon peeled and minced fresh ginger

• 2 scallions, both white and green parts, thinly sliced, divided

• 1½ pounds boneless, skinless chicken thighs

• Sesame seeds, for garnish

Directions:

1. In the electric pressure cooker, combine the tamari, pineapple, brown sugar, garlic, ginger, and white parts of the scallions. Dip the chicken thighs in the sauce to coat all sides, then nestle each piece in the sauce in a single layer.

2. Close and lock the lid of the pressure cooker. Set the valve to sealing.

 3. Cook on high pressure for 15 minutes.

4. When the cooking is complete, hit Cancel and quick release the pressure.

5. Once the pin drops, unlock and remove the lid.

6. Hit Sauté and simmer until the sauce has thickened and is the consistency you like, about 5

 minutes. Hit Cancel. Shred or chop the chicken, if desired.

7. Remove the chicken to serving plates or a platter, sprinkle with the green parts of the scallions and sesame seeds. Serve immediately.

8. Nutrition Info: Per serving: Calories: 214; Total Fat: 6g; Protein: 30g; Carbohydrates: 9g; Sugars: 6g; Fiber: 1g; Sodium: 540mg

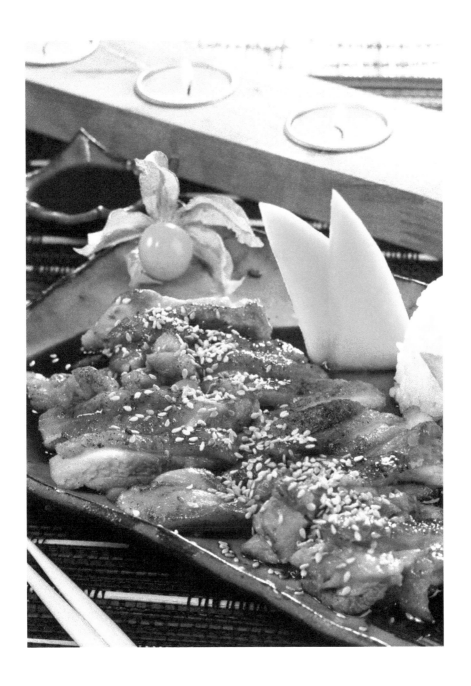

Zucchini With Tomatoes

Servings: 8

Cooking Time: 11 Minutes

Ingredients:

• 6 medium zucchinis, chopped roughly

• 1 pound cherry tomatoes

• 2 small onions, chopped roughly

• 2 tablespoons fresh basil, chopped

• 1 cup water

• 1 tablespoon olive oil

• 2 garlic cloves, minced

• Salt and ground black pepper, as required

Directions:

1. In the Pressure Pot, place oil and press "Sauté". Now add the onion, garlic, ginger, and spices and cook for about 3-4 minutes.

2. Add the zucchinis and tomatoes and cook for about 1-minutes.

3. Press "Cancel" and stir in the remaining ingredients except basil.

4. Close the lid and place the pressure valve to "Seal" position.

5. Press "Manual" and cook under "High Pressure" for about minutes.

6. Press "Cancel" and allow a "Natural" release.

7. Open the lid and transfer the vegetable mixture onto a serving platter.

8. Garnish with basil and serve.

9. Nutrition Info: Per serving: Calories: 57, Fats: 2.1g, Carbs: , Sugar: 4.8g, Proteins: 2.5g, Sodium: 39mg

Lightning Source UK Ltd.
Milton Keynes UK
UKHW020624190721
387392UK00001B/9

9 781803 424095